Healthiest Sick Person I Know

Marsha Nixon Powell

Copyright © 2024 Marsha Nixon Powell
All rights reserved
First Edition

Fulton Books
Meadville, PA

Published by Fulton Books 2024

ISBN 979-8-89221-110-9 (paperback)
ISBN 979-8-89221-111-6 (digital)

Printed in the United States of America

This book is dedicated to my family and in loving memory of my mother, Betty and my sister, Brenda.

ACKNOWLEDGMENTS

To my daughters: Qiana and Cierra, and my grandson, Mark: my love and appreciation for keeping me grounded and focused and encouraging me to remain positive and to be the best that I can be.

CHAPTER 1

I'm Here! The Formative Years

I was born Marsha Jean Nixon on March 1, 1950, at Thomas Jefferson University Hospital in downtown Philadelphia, Pennsylvania. I lived a good life with my mother, Betty, and my sister, Brenda in Richard Allen Homes housing projects in North Philadelphia, one of the first housing projects in Philadelphia, built in 1941 and named after Richard Allen, founder of the African Methodist Episcopal Church. It was demolished in 1996 to make way for updated single-family dwellings, but for some of us, the Richard Allen Homes housing project will always be home. I don't recall my father growing up, due to the fact that my mother and father divorced early in my life. Even though I didn't know my father, I did know my paternal family—a large family known as the Deveros and Nixons who lived in North Philadelphia. My father was adopted by his biological aunt (his mother's sister), so my aunt was my grandmother, and my grandmother was my aunt. I know, clear as mud. Also, my mother and her sister (my aunt Letha) were married to brothers—my father, Leroy, and my uncle Herman, so my first cousins and I are double cousins. My father was close to both of his mothers, I learned, which sounds strange but was normal for my family. My mother worked at Nalor Knitting Factory in the center city area, I believe as a seamstress. My sister and I were pretty much on our own after school until my mother came home. Times were different then; you constantly had nosy neighbors, family members, and close friends keeping an eye on you. Sometimes we went to our grandmother's house after school and spent time playing with our cousins. My grandmother also lived in Richard Allen Homes close to East Poplar Playground, near Eighth and Poplar Streets. During the fifties and sixties—I know this sounds hard to believe—but television during that time had only three stations: ABC, CBS, and NBC, and the TVs went off the air around 12:00 a.m. and played the "Star-Spangled Banner" when it came back on in the morning. My favorite shows were the after-school cartoons and shows with Sally Starr, showing *Popeye*, *The Three Stooges*, and Disney shows with the Mickey Mouse Club featuring the Mouseketeers with Annette Funicello, Darlene Gillespie, Cubby O'Brien, and the many other talented Disney actors. On Saturdays, I watched my favorite westerns—*The Rifleman*, *Bonanza*, and *Gunsmoke*. I'm still watching and enjoying the shows on TV now. Even though I lived in North Philly, I had many relatives who lived in South Philly (Point Breeze area). I attended New Central Baptist Church at Twenty-Third and Lombard Streets, where I was a Sunday school teacher, also played the piano for the children in Sunday school, and participated in the Wee Folk Music/Piano Recitals. We also attended St. Paul's Baptist Church located in North Philadelphia at Tenth and Wallace Streets. Also, years ago, we used to attend the MET (Metropolitan Opera House) at Broad and Poplar Streets, in North Philadelphia, which was a church officiated by the great preacher and evangelist, the Reverend Thea Jones, which was one of the early mega churches with over one thousand members and a two-hundred-voice choir led by Barry Currington, a flamboyant choirmaster.

    I attended the neighborhood elementary school of John Hancock, in

I'm the Healthiest Sick Person I Know

North Philadelphia, located at Twelfth and Fairmount Avenues. Many of the teachers during this period (Mr. Young/Mr. Jones) were true disciplinarians and used yardsticks to deliver corporate punishment on your hand or sometimes on your backside and many times came to your home after school to inform your parents if you misbehaved or were truant during school time. Before there was school busing in Philadelphia, I was able to identify with teenager Chris Rock's experiences growing up in from *Everybody Hates Chris* sitcom series. I had to get up early in the morning to catch three different public transportation vehicles—former Philadelphia Transportation Company or PTC (the name before SEPTA), catching the 23 trolley at Eleventh and Fairmount Avenues, then the elevated train at Eleventh and Market Streets, then getting off at Fifty-Sixth and Market Streets, and then catching the G bus to Shaw Junior High School (now called middle schools) at Fifty-Fourth and Warrington Avenues in Southwest Philly. Then at the end of the school day, back home again—each way over one and a half hours. I remember one time when there was a transportation strike—no end seemed to be in sight. I had to catch the commuter train (from Seventeenth and JFK Boulevard in center city) to school. (I don't remember how I got to center city. I guess I walked.). Somehow along the way, I lost my train ticket and had to walk all the way from Southwest Philly to my home in North Philly. The walk was well over six hours long in the dead of winter—January 1963. You best believe I never lost my train ticket again. When I graduated from Shaw Junior High School, I was used to traveling the distance each day, but the Philadelphia School District reversed their ruling that you could not go to high school out your district, so I was unable to attend the high school I

I'm the Healthiest Sick Person I Know

wanted to go to—which was Overbrook High School in Southwest Philadelphia.

I have early memories of attending R & B concerts at the Uptown Theatre at Broad and Susquehanna/Dauphin Streets hosted by the greatest DJ on the radio at the time—Georgie Woods, of Philadelphia Radio Station WDAS, who has a street named after him in North Philly. Some of the best entertainers performed at the Uptown, such as Smokey Robinson & The Miracles, Ray Charles, The Jackson 5, Patti LaBelle, and The Temptations, to name a few. I had the best time seeing them perform live.

In 1964, I attended the William Penn High School for Girls, which was my neighborhood high school located in North Philadelphia at Fifteenth and Wallace Streets. What a change. I was able to walk to school. In spite of being disappointed because I was not able to attend Overbrook High School, I thoroughly enjoyed attending William Penn.

I was a well-rounded student, being a member of the Future Teachers of America Club, the Spanish Club, and the swimming team. At the time, Benjamin Franklin High School was right around the corner, and I'm sure not a lot of people remember that Benjamin Franklin used to be an all-boys' school. Ben Franklin was our kindred school. We attended their football and basketball games and cheered for their teams at home and away. Even though it has been over fifty-five years, I still have lifelong friends that I meet with socially on a regular basis. During my last six months at William Penn, my mother remarried, and we moved from Richard Allen Homes in North Philly to the area of Eighteenth and Cheltenham Avenues in West Oak Lane. Here I go ago traveling from one end of town to the other. Senior year flew by. We went on our class trip to New York City. We had lunch at Tavern-on-the Green and danced all evening at the Cheetah

I'm the Healthiest Sick Person I Know

Night Club, one of the most famous discotheque clubs during that time in Manhattan, New York. One of my fondest memories from high school was my high school prom. I had a preprom dinner the night before along with eight of my friends and their dates. My mother was a very good seamstress who made matching Easter outfits for me and my sister along with Sunday dress-up outfits. My mother designed my gold prom gown, and it was beautiful! Our prom was at the Mark IV Ball Room on City Avenue in Bala Cynwyd, Pennsylvania, and we enjoyed dancing to the upbeat music of "The Happening!" sung by The Supremes and slow danced to "You're My Everything" sung by The Temptations. Afterward, six of us (three couples) drove to Atlantic City (precasinos) and had a great time until on the way back, we had a car accident on the Atlantic City Expressway. Fortunately, no one was seriously hurt. I graduated from William Penn High School

(Torch 67) in 1967. Graduation day was very memorable. I remember crossing the stage full of pride and receiving my diploma knowing I was entering a new phase of my life along with seeing the loving and proud looks on my family's faces.

CHAPTER 2

Information Operator — What's That?

After high school, I was hired and worked as an information operator for the Bell Telephone Company of Philadelphia on Arch Street in downtown Philadelphia, which later became the present Verizon Company. The position, which was also called directory assistance, entailed answering phone calls from people calling in who needed phone numbers and street addresses for residential and business customers. While working at Bell Telephone, the information operators used the White Pages and Yellow Pages (pre–

cell phones) which were combined in one big reference tome. It was one of the strictest and most stressful companies I ever worked for. During work time, if you wanted to take a bathroom break or leave for lunch, you had to put a light on at your work station to ask for permission to leave, because someone had to fill in for you. Of course, sometimes you were not able to leave right away, because the replacement person had not yet returned from either their break or lunch. But at a young age (seventeen), I learned a lot about diverse people and personalities in a business environment. I also learned discipline, attending work on time and daily, and also realized that it wasn't the job for me! During this time, I believe 1968, I was involved in another strike—the Bell Telephone Union Company Strike. Since I had not joined the union, and being young and innocent at that time to working relationships, I didn't know you were not supposed to cross the picket

I'm the Healthiest Sick Person I Know

line. I was threatened by the union workers, which caused me to be afraid to enter my place of employment, and was also called a scab! During this time, a friend I knew from the Southwest area asked me to go on his high school prom, ironically, at, of all places, Overbrook Senior High School. My employers would not allow me to leave work early to attend, so I had to get completely dressed at work, and I got to wear my gold gown again, and in my formal wear and donning my tiara, I was picked up outside of my place of employment. In spite of it all, I had a great time that night, but that was the final straw as far as working at Bell Telephone.

After making a decision not to attend college, due to high financial costs and tuition, I decided to attend business/executive secretary school at the Philadelphia School of Business Office Training at Seventeenth and Chestnut Streets in center city Philadelphia. To bring back longtime memories, I took the following courses—English, typing (manual typewriter), and Gregg shorthand/dictation and using a Dictaphone. I was able to type 80 words per minute (wpm) and took dictation at 100 wpm. The coursework was very demanding, but the young women who attended were very supportive of each other, along with the teachers, who were very helpful and encouraged the students to be as successful and professional as possible, as we prepared to enter into the business environment. After graduating from business school, I was initially employed as a legal secretary at the Philadelphia National Bank in their legal department in downtown Philadelphia and then eventually became a longtime employee at First Pennsylvania Bank at Fifteenth and Market Streets in the Centre Square Building, as an executive assistant for over ten years. I truly enjoyed that job. At that time, the dress code was truly business professional, with no casual Fridays or work-at-home opportuni-

I'm the Healthiest Sick Person I Know

ties. I also met my future husband, Richard, who worked there as a loan officer.

When most workers went to the job cafeteria or to the nearby restaurants for lunch, my girlfriend and I went to the bowling lanes (Center City Bowling Lanes) near the Greyhound Bus Terminal at Seventeenth and Markets Streets and bowled, ate our lunch, and then rushed from the bowling lanes to make it back to work on time. When I didn't brown bag it in the cafeteria, we would sometimes have lunch at Howard Johnson's, Horn & Hardart, or White Tower Hamburgers (great grilled burgers and thick delicious malted milkshakes—before becoming dominated by fast food restaurants).

During this time, there are so many good memories that I can remember, because after I would get off work, I would walk around downtown Philly area and shop at such department stores as: Strawbridge & Clothiers, Wanamaker's, Gimbels, and my favorite five-and-dime—Grant's, which had the best grilled hot dogs. Sometimes on Sundays after church, my sister and I would go to the Penny Arcade and take photos, and if we had enough change leftover, we would go to Horn & Hardart's Food automart, also located in Center City. I can't go without mentioning one of the most popular eateries—the sidewalk food carts that sold the Philly famous cheesesteaks and salted pretzels with mustard—true Philadelphian—or cheese. During the summer, an Italian ice was the best way to beat the heat. I didn't know what owning a car was—I went everywhere on the bus, trolley, subway or elevated train, or walked.

As a young person, for entertainment and fun, we went to the neighborhood bowling lanes, Lynnewood Lanes, and the neighborhood movie theatre—Erlen Theatre, both located in West Oak Lane, which have both since closed many years ago. There was also one of the best hoagie shops—Lee's Hoagies on Cheltenham Avenue. When anyone would visit me, you best believe we went there for sandwiches and sodas. There were also other early restaurants and pre-fast-food restaurants, such as Roy Rogers, Howard Johnsons, Bob's Big Boy, and the Stenton Diner. We also went shopping at the two major malls—Cheltenham Mall and Cedarbrook Mall. It was fun shopping at Kmart and Gimbels—years ago two of the many delightful places to shop throughout the years, especially during holidays.

CHAPTER 3

Married/Family Life

After meeting Richard at work, we dated for about one year and then married in January of 1977. We had a good relationship, but I was a little on the flirty side, and Richard warned me several times about flirting with other guys. I promised that I would stop (fingers crossed behind my back). So one day, while we were waiting on the platform to get on the subway, a man approached me, and I began talking with him. Richard had just walked away, but turned back around once he saw me laughing and talking as usual and was about ready to step to the gentleman. I stopped him in time and explained that he

I'm the Healthiest Sick Person I Know

was my uncle Marvin and introduced him to my father's younger brother. We had a good laugh about it.

A year and a half after we were married, we had a beautiful daughter, Qiana Crystal. Qiana was a beautiful baby with the biggest and brightest brown eyes. We had a good marriage, and we used to travel to Baltimore, Maryland, on a regular basis to visit my in-laws. My husband, Richard, has a big family in Baltimore, Maryland, and in Philadelphia—the Powells. We had fun times over the years, visiting and partying with his grandparents—Dorothy and Curt, aunts, uncles, brothers and sisters, and a host of cousins. He also had two young sons—one in Baltimore (Ricky) and one in Pleasantville, New Jersey (Hakim). We also had fun times with my family in Philly during the holidays—my favorite holidays were Thanksgiving and Christmas. We rotated having Thanksgiving and Christmas at my mother's house with my stepfather, Fred, my sister's place with her two daughters, Jawana and Justine, and then at my place. Those were the best times—we always had a houseful of family and friends. Eating, watching the football games, listening to music, and dancing was a regular holiday ritual. And the best dessert of all times—sweet potato pie with whipped cream or vanilla ice cream.

After about two years of marriage, around 1979, Richard, Qiana and I relocated to San Diego, California, and lived there for seven years. It was very frightening since it was my first time flying, being a new mother, and we didn't really know anyone in California. My husband was hired as a vice president at Crocker Bank, and I was employed as an administrative assistant at the same bank (but not working for him). We lived in a beautiful area of San Diego called Point Loma, not far from Coronado Beach and near the San Diego International

Airport. My mother and stepfather came out to visit several times, and also my sister along with her two daughters, came out to visit from time to time. While living in San Diego, I got to visit, San Francisco, Las Vegas, and Tijuana, Mexico. My girlfriends from Philadelphia also came to visit us. One of my best birthdays was when my girlfriend and her daughter came to visit, and we drove from San Diego to Las Vegas across the hot desert. We encountered all kinds of obstacles along the way—wind, heavy rains, and unruly truck drivers—but we made it there and had a great time.

Unfortunately, I was not happy living in California, and my daughter and me moved back to Philadelphia. My husband and I separated, and eventually we divorced. After I moved back to Philly, I decided to exert my independence after finding work as an executive assistant, and I decided to purchase my first home by myself for me and my daughter. We had to get familiar with living back in Philadelphia again. My daughter was seven years old, and it became the first time that she experienced playing in the snow.

I worked as an executive assistant/office administrator at CIGNA Corporation for more than fifteen years at One Liberty Plaza and Two Liberty Plaza on the fifty-third floor and fifty-fifth floors, respectively. My daughter was accepted and attended Philadelphia High School for Girls and graduated with a full four-year scholarship to Pennsylvania State University at the main campus in State College, Pennsylvania. She was only sixteen when she moved away from home to attend college for the first time. Surprisingly, she adapted very well. After receiving her bachelor of science degree in computer engineering, she attended Morgan State University in Baltimore, Maryland. During that time, I went to college and graduated from Peirce College in Philadelphia with a bachelor of science degree in business administration (at the age of fifty-two) while working full-time, and my daughter received her master's degree from Morgan State University the same year in 2002 (still receiving a full scholarship).

My time at CIGNA was a great developing and learning experience. I worked in the Diversity Department for the vice president as an administrative assistant who was the best supervisor, and then later I was promoted to the position of office manager in the finance department, reporting to the vice president, who was the manager overseeing a staff of more than thirty employees. I had the opportunity to travel to several of CIGNA's locations—Bloomfield and Hartford, Connecticut, and Atlanta, Georgia, to name a few of the locations.

CIGNA had the best training and career opportunities. When I attended Peirce College, it was entirely funded by CIGNA. They also had the best company benefits—401(k) and pension plan, and healthcare benefits along with family leave options. During my time at CIGNA, when I was diagnosed with cancer and during my hospital stay in the hospital, along with the many medications I had to take, thankfully, I incurred minimal out-of-pocket expenses.

CHAPTER 4

We Had Good Times/ The Ladies of WP67

I truly enjoyed myself being back in Philly. My family, including my mother, stepfather, and sister enjoyed bowling at Washington Lanes in the West Oak Lane/Stenton area of Philadelphia. Washington Lanes closed many years ago, but I am sure along with myself, many others recall the fun we had bowling at the Lanes, which the local newspapers described as being the "loudest bowling lane in Philadelphia." There were forty lanes in the house—twenty on one side and twenty on the other side. During the late 1980s, we bowled competitively. The league was named Travelers Bowling League—even though we didn't travel anywhere. My mother was the treasurer for many years, which was very detailed and involved. She had to collect the money from the captains on the leagues and deposit the money in the bank—CoreStates Bank—throughout the season and then collect the funds at the end of the bowling season and distribute the funds based on a team bowling prize fund that was voted on by the president of the league, team captains, and bowling team members and paid to the bowlers based on the winning teams from the top to the bottom. There were also money prizes paid to individuals based on their top winning scores. After my mother retired from being the treasurer, she passed the torch to me. I was also the treasurer for many years.

As the teams bowled, there was a speakeasy going on at the bowling lanes in the downstairs area called the Blue Room. As we

I'm the Healthiest Sick Person I Know

bowled, one of the bowlers would call out over the loudspeaker, "The Blue Room is open." The bowlers knew that that meant it was time for beer and spirits. I think it made us bowl better. There were some of the best bowlers that I remember: males—Charlie J. and Gordon. I was also definitely impressed by the female bowlers: Micki, Marion, and Joyce. And of course, there were others. We also had music piped in in the downstairs area. It was very similar to a club-like atmosphere except without having to pay a cover charge.

There were also other bowling lanes throughout the Philadelphia area (which have since closed): Adams Lanes, Stenton Lanes, and Boulevard Lanes, which offered a variety of bowling options: senior leagues, teachers leagues, juniors leagues, mixed leagues, and Special Olympics leagues. Many of the local high schools sponsored leagues for the students as an after-school activity to promote fun, fair play, competition, and sportsmanship. After school, parents always knew where their children were. There were also bus trips from Adams Lanes to the casinos in Atlantic City. Again, good times. Unfortunately, many of the bowling lanes have closed, and competitive team bowling is a dying sport. But many of us have fond memories of past bowling times and the many friends and close relationships that were developed. There were also generations of families who bowled and passed along the love and competitiveness of bowling down to their children and grandchildren. My daughter not only bowled at Washington Lanes but was also employed during the summers as a cashier. My grandson bowled at Thunderbird Lanes on Castor Avenue in Northeast Philadelphia as a member of the Special Olympics Team, which included a complete reenactment of the Special Olympics Games.

I'm the Healthiest Sick Person I Know

After bowling, many of the bowlers went out to eat at Stenton Diner, or sometimes to the Mt. Airy Lodge, or Limekiln Pike Bar for more drinking and dancing, and maybe sometimes back to Washington Lanes again for more bowling.

There were more fun and enjoyable times. My stepfather (who was a supervisor) and my sister (who was employed for many years as a bus driver and subway cashier) both worked for the Southeastern Transportation Company (SEPTA), which as I mentioned earlier is the transportation company for Philadelphia and the suburbs. SEPTA had monthly cabarets (parties at ballrooms), overnight trips to Montreal, Canada, and bowling and holiday parties on the Spirit of Philadelphia. We were able to have great fun, along with dancing, drinking, and eating food in a safe environment at reasonable prices.

As I mentioned earlier, I attended William Penn High School for Girls and graduated in 1967. William Penn became coed, but moved from its original location, to Broad Street in the Temple University area and has since closed permanently. This seems so strange since William Penn founded the province of Pennsylvania in 1681 and is also a statute that stands atop city hall in center city Philadelphia. Thanks to social media, many of my classmates have been able to locate one another and remain in touch. We have a group of ladies—the Ladies of WP67—that talk socially on Zoom calls and meet on a regular basis for dinner and drinks at Gallo's Restaurant in Northeast Philadelphia, which plays the best Motown music, to talk about what we are up to, our health, families, and a little gossip. We make sure to include prayer, motivational input, and positive thoughts during our gatherings. Since we no longer have a formal student administration, we put

I'm the Healthiest Sick Person I Know

together a Chit Chat, Chew & Chug gathering to celebrate our class reunion in 1997 at a friend's house. Even one of our teachers attended. It was small but cozy and fun.

In 2006, four of us got together and went on the Tom Joyner Fantastic Voyage Cruise aboard the *Navigator* of the Seas Royal Caribbean Royal Ship in Caribbean, which is the largest "African American Party with A Purpose Cruise," and went to several Caribbean islands—Cuba, Jamaica, and Puerto Rico. I had such a good time on board that I never really left the ship when we visited the different ports. There was live R & B, soul, funk, and gospel music, legendary music performers, such as Maze featuring Frankie Beverly and Bobby Brown, along with island hopping and twenty-four-hour food and drinks. One of the entertainers on the ship summed it up best when he said, "The whole world needs to come on a Tom Joyner cruise to learn how to love one another." Great people of the older persuasion were in attendance and thoroughly enjoyed themselves. Not only is the cruise fun and entertaining, it is a one-of-a kind celebration that supports students at historically black colleges and universities (HBCUs) for over more than twenty years and is still going on even though Tom Joyner has retired and is no longer on the radio.

God willing, we plan to meet and greet at Gallo's and stay in touch as long as we are able to and hopefully, may go on another Tom Joyner Fantastic Voyage Cruise together again.

I'm the Healthiest Sick Person I Know

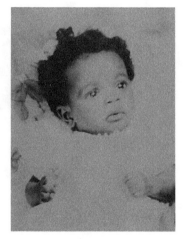

Me at six months old

Marsha Nixon Powell

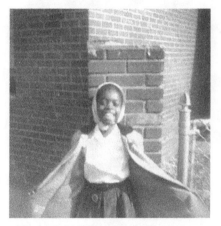

When I lived at Richard Allen Homes

I'm the Healthiest Sick Person I Know

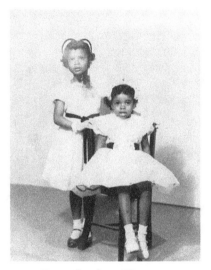

Easter Sunday - My sister,
Brenda and me

Marsha Nixon Powell

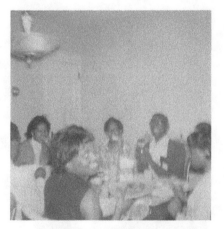

Pre-prom Dinner

I'm the Healthiest Sick Person I Know

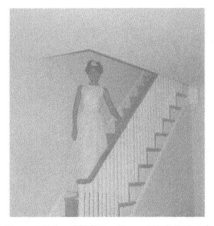

Prom Night - William Penn High School

Marsha Nixon Powell

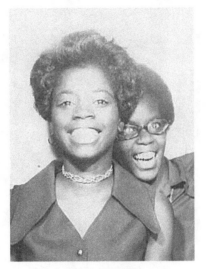

Me and my girlfriend, Brenda,
at the Penny Arcade

I'm the Healthiest Sick Person I Know

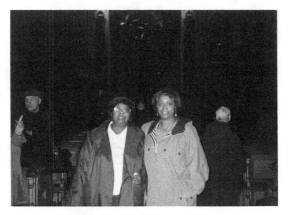

Mom and me in Montreal, Canada

Marsha Nixon Powell

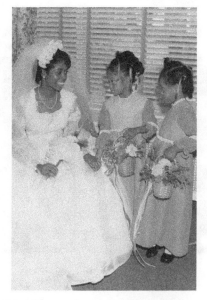

Me with my nieces - Jawana and Justine

I'm the Healthiest Sick Person I Know

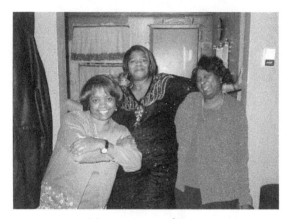

Me, my sister and mom

Marsha Nixon Powell

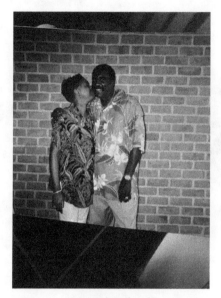

Me and Richard

I'm the Healthiest Sick Person I Know

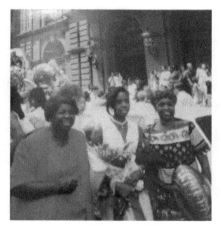

My mom, my daughter, Qiana, and me Girls' High Graduation

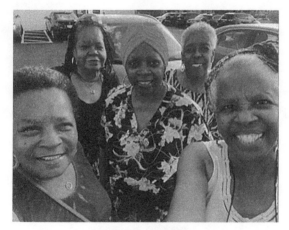

The Ladies of WP67

I'm the Healthiest Sick Person I Know

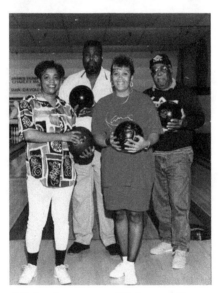

My bowling team at Washington Lanes

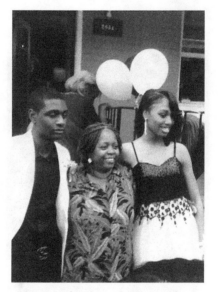

Me, my daughter, Cierra, and her prom date - Northeast High School

I'm the Healthiest Sick Person I Know

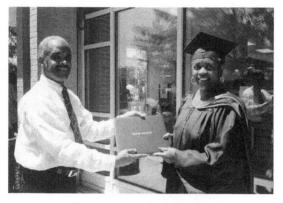

CJ and me at my graduation
from Peirce College

Marsha Nixon Powell

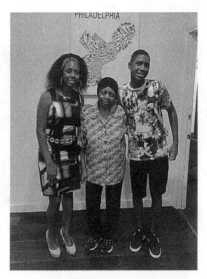

Me, my daughter, Qiana,
and my grandson, Mark

CHAPTER 5

Day Care/Foster Care

My life took a change when I was laid off from CIGNA and decided to start my own business. I started a family-based day care at my home on Eastwood Street in Northeast Philadelphia. During this time, I became a grandmother for the first time to my handsome grandson, Mark. I was also a foster mother to more than six children throughout the years and became a legal guardian/mom to my other beautiful daughter, Cierra. I hadn't had young children at my home in several years, so it was a whole new experience to have the responsibility of raising children again. I initially opened my home to three children—two biological sisters and one brother. Even though you love them and know you will miss them, the main objective of being a foster parent is to hopefully reunite them with their biological parent(s) or close family member(s) (possibly grandparent or older sibling). Being a foster mother taught me patience and endurance and above all, love for another person's child(ren).

In order to become a foster parent, you need to be ready to be thoroughly investigated by local, state, and federal agencies—such as having to complete the FBI clearance, child abuse clearance, and criminal history clearance. It would also be helpful to take a training course in CPR and first aid to receive certifications. One stipulation that has changed over the years—you can be a single foster parent without an age stipulation; just be healthy mentally, emotionally, and physically. First and foremost, you should have a loving and caring home that is void

I'm the Healthiest Sick Person I Know

of bias/prejudice and without any prejudgments. Ironically, the foster care agency—JJC (Juvenile Justice Center of Philadelphia in Germantown, Pennsylvania), who placed the children in my home, is the same agency I currently work for as a behavioral health technician (BHT) for the Philadelphia School District.

As I mentioned earlier, I also opened up my home as a childcare provider and owner/operator of "For Your Kids" Family Day Care in Northeast Philadelphia. I opened my day care in the city of Philadelphia, which offered an abundance of helpful information to assist with licensing, zoning approval, inspections, etc. in order to begin starting and running your day care business. In order to prevent a lot of heartache, one of the first things you should do is put together a contract between parents and providers (parent handbook) to inform the parents of such things as the daily schedule (opening and closing times) what you will provide, daily care that will be given, and what is expected of the parent/guardian—for example, when fees should be paid and the times children should be dropped off and picked up. I was the chief cook and bottle washer. Basically, I was the sole caregiver (for four to six children).

I provided breakfast, lunch, and snacks daily. Part of the regular schedule was free play (trips to the playground) and planned activities (story and reading times, visits to the local library, and also during the summer, walks to the park and the neighborhood swimming pool). I provided care for infants and children, five and under, along with after-school care for children up to the age of eleven or twelve. The neighborhood elementary school was two blocks away and was one of the better elementary schools in the area—S. Solis-Cohen Elementary School. My day care initially started off with family members and close friends, but favorable feedback helped my day care to develop and grow with new parents.

A few years after I started the day care in my home—For Your Kids Family Day Care, my grandson, Mark, was diagnosed with autism around the age of four. After watching my grandson go through being diagnosed by his pediatrician (Dr. McLaughlin), receiving early intervention, and the training he received in special education classes in school from the special education teachers and the therapeutic staff support (TSS), encouraged me to apply for training and become a school-based behavioral health technician (BHT). I thoroughly enjoyed being a childcare provider and business owner, but after over ten years of working as a childcare provider, I closed my day care and began working for the Philadelphia School District in the Northeast Philadelphia area for the public and charter schools as a behavioral health technician (BHT).

CHAPTER 6

BHT/Substitute Teaching—Chosen Career Paths

After over more than ten years, I closed my Family Day Care and have been working for the past five years as a behavioral health technician (BHT) for the Philadelphia School District.

I have worked one-on-one with children with behavioral diagnoses such as ADHD and autism. I have also provided support in-home, community, and school settings. Like many people that work in this field, many have close family members that have dealt with behavioral and emotional problems. I have over ten years of personal and five years of professional experience working with special-needs children. As you work with teachers and special-needs children in the school environment, you become aware there are so many short-term and long-term goals and achievements that need to be followed and met by the behavioral health technician along with the supervisor—behavior consultant (BC)—who supports and consults with you to assist with crisis prevention and management.

Again, as working with foster children, there are many credentials that a behavioral health technician has to meet—child abuse, criminal, FBI clearance—being fingerprinted as a Pennsylvania DHS Child Care Services employee, and you are considered an employee who is mandated to report child abuse if observed or perceived. You also must take training in cardiopulmonary resuscitation (CPR)/automated external defibrillation (AED) adults and child and first aid to receive certifications. You must also have yearly physical and tuberculosis (TB) tests.

The behavioral health technician is there to assist the child with managing his/her behavior in a safe and appropriate manner on a one-to-one basis. The overall responsibility of the behavioral health technician is to provide one-to-one therapeutic/behavioral support and behavioral interventions to children/adolescents in home, school and/or community settings in order to help the client achieve goals identified on their treatment plan.

I enjoy the opportunity of working with the children and continue to learn and experience new things myself constantly. I am asked this question on a regular basis: what do you have to do to work with special needs children? There is no cookie-cutter answer—

no child or diagnosis is the same. Each child is unique in their own way.

I have observed over the past years and have also noted on the news that there is a shortage of teachers in the Philadelphia school system. There is an abundance of problems due to pay, working conditions, lack of support, and many of the teachers going to the suburbs, and also many of the teachers leaving the profession. I have decided to try and pursue a possible career working as a substitute teacher in the Philadelphia School District. I also look forward, if the opportunity presents itself, to a possible career working as a special education teacher.

CHAPTER 7

1, 2, 3 Punch

I have been diagnosed/treated with several medical conditions over the past twenty-five years—stage 2 ovarian cancer at the age of forty-five, heart murmur/irregular heartbeat, hypertension (high blood pressure), and high cholesterol. I suffered a TIA (mini stroke), type 2 diabetes, stage 3 chronic kidney disease, Achilles Tendonitis, laser eye surgery, and a slip and fall in August of 2022 and recently endured a root canal.

In 1995, I was diagnosed with type 2 ovarian cancer after dealing with moderate to severe ongoing pain that took over a year to discover. I was given several different diag-

I'm the Healthiest Sick Person I Know

noses, from going through the change of life to gastric stomach ulcer, which also involved several trips to the doctor and emergency wards.

After enduring excruciating pain that felt like at times going through childbirth along with heavy bleeding, I was recommended by my doctor to schedule an ultrasound to see if that would help with a diagnosis. Two days before I was scheduled for the ultrasound, the pains started again, and I went to the emergency ward straight from bowling. After the doctors ran several tests, you can imagine my surprise when the doctor said, "Let me cut to the chase" and told me he believed I had some form of cancer and to follow up with my family doctor. Two of my friends were there with me, and we were all opened-mouthed and stunned, to say the least. Long story short, I had exploratory surgery to remove a tumor (complete hysterectomy), also stayed in the cancer ward for over a week at Abington Memorial Hospital in Abington, Pennsylvania, and received six treatments of chemotherapy. My daughter, Qiana, had just started college at Penn State, Main Campus in State College, Pennsylvania, and she was away from home. I didn't want her to miss classes so early in the semester, so I held off telling her for a while. Luckily, I had family and friends willing to pitch in and help me at home and take me for my appointments to the doctor (pre rideshare). Unfortunately, I had a recurrence a year later, with additional treatments of chemo, but thank God I have been cancer-free for over twenty-five years. Sadly, I learned that approximately twenty-five thousand women in the United States are diagnosed with this disease each year and possibly fourteen thousand women will die from this disease in the US.

Along with the severe medical conditions and psychological fear of having a diagnosis of ovarian cancer has impacted my life

I'm the Healthiest Sick Person I Know

in several ways. I believe that I developed ovarian cancer due to the prolonged use of talc powder. The major seller of this product has stopped selling talc-based baby powder in the United States. I have been tested for family genetic traits of ovarian cancer—none displayed. There are more than sixteen thousand lawsuits from consumers claiming the talc powder has caused their cancer. The lawsuits allege that the company's talc products have been contaminated with asbestos, a known carcinogen (substances that may increase your risk of cancer).

During the past several years, I have been diagnosed with chronic high blood pressure (family genetic problem)—which unfortunately many times does not exhibit any symptoms—heart murmur/irregular heartbeat, high cholesterol, which led to my undergoing a TIA (transient ischemic attack, also known as a "mini stroke"). Again, I did not exhibit any previous medical or physical symptoms. I was working as a caregiver at a nursing home in Langhorne, Bucks County, Pennsylvania, and sat down to take my break—this was during the 2016 Presidential Election (Hilary Clinton and Donald Trump)—and woke up later in St. Mary's Center Hospital in Langhorne, Pennsylvania. I don't remember anything prior to or immediately after, but I am fully recovered and have no permanent damage to my brain or body. I also have been diagnosed with type 2 diabetes (another genetic family disease), which has ultimately caused me to be diagnosed with stage 3 chronic kidney disease (CKD3). Since I have been diagnosed with chronic kidney disease, I have discovered that several family members have also been diagnosed with many of the same medical conditions that I have. We are all supportive of each other. I have a very knowledgeable and well-informed medical provider at the Excel Medical Center who has kept me well advised

I'm the Healthiest Sick Person I Know

of my medical conditions, and I make sure to follow up and keep my appointments and take my meds in a timely manner.

As I will continue to emphasize, when faced with ongoing medical conditions, please try to remain positive, keep your appointments, take your meds, don't hesitate to ask your doctor any questions regarding your diagnosis and treatments. Also, follow your doctor's orders, along with surrounding yourself with positive and supporting family and friends.

Around 2017, I became the caregiver for my mother, who was diagnosed with high blood pressure and stage 3 chronic kidney disease, which later progressed to stage 5 renal (kidney) failure. I was her caregiver for almost three years, and being able to take care of my mother in her home brought me joy and peace. In June of 2020, she was placed in home hospice care. It allowed me time to bind with her and gave me the strength needed to assist her with her declining health. My mother succumbed to renal (end life) kidney disease in November of 2020 a week before Thanksgiving at the age of ninety. Even though it was a very sad time for me, I was thankful and grateful to be able to be there with my mother at her peaceful demise.

My sister, who lived in Charlotte, North Carolina, initially was not going to be able to come back to Philadelphia for our mother's funeral, due to the chronic ailments that she endured—she was type 1 diabetic and took insulin daily, was on daily oxygen due to breathing problems, and sometimes she had difficulty with walking. She was able to drive the distance by car, which was over ten hours away to Philadelphia for the homegoing services. My mother was an avid bowler before her illness, and she was a longtime member and usher at Second Pilgrim Baptist Church in North Philadelphia.

In spite of her health, I was pleased my sister and my nieces and nephews were able make it to Philly for the services. Unfortunately, and sadly, my sister also passed away a month later on Christmas Day (which was her favorite holiday to spend with her grandchildren), due to complications from COVID-19 and type 1 diabetes at the age of seventy-two.

I love and miss my mother and sister very much.

CHAPTER 8

The Aftermath— No Matter What

My grandson, Mark, recently graduated from Samuel Fels High School in Northeast Philadelphia, earning high honors and is preparing for technical training in the hopes of being employed as an IT/support/computer technician. After all his hard work and dedication, I was so proud to see him walk across the stage in his cap and gown.

In spite of my many medical conditions, I feel relatively healthy, upbeat, positive, and in good spirits. I make sure to follow up with my doctor's instructions and keep my medical appointments and take my meds as directed. Also, as I mentioned, I am a twenty-five-year cancer survivor. After I was diagnosed with ovarian cancer—which involved staying in Abington Memorial Hospital for over a week—I had a complete hysterectomy at the age of forty-five and six treatments of chemotherapy. Unfortunately, there were so many side effects from the chemo treatments—loss of hair and appetite, nausea—which caused me to endure drastic weight loss. My hair loss was devastating because my hair fell out almost immediately after the first chemo treatment. I didn't want to seem vain, but losing your hair messes with your self-esteem, because it not only happened once but twice—all over my head, eyebrows, etc. Thank goodness for turbans and wigs of various styles and textures, and my hair did eventually grow back.

After my surgery (complete hysterectomy), I was able to see the humor—didn't have to worry about tampons or monthly cramps anymore. I had a recurrence a year later, but I am currently cancer-free.

As I mentioned, I have been recently diagnosed with chronic kidney disease stage 3 (CKD 3), which cannot be reversed or cured. I can only try to slow the progression so it won't progress to stage 4 kidney failure or stage 5 renal kidney disease, which will result in daily dialysis or a kidney transplant. Many people may have this disease, but are totally unaware because the symptoms are initially mild. Kidney disease means your kidneys aren't working properly and are beginning to lose their function. Chronic kidney disease worsens over time. High blood pressure and diabetes (which I have both medical conditions) are two common causes of chronic kidney disease. Also, it can be a genetic condition (which my mother was diagnosed with). Unfortunately, it cannot be reversed or cured, and will progress to stage 4 or stage

I'm the Healthiest Sick Person I Know

5, and dialysis or kidney transplant will be needed. It is not necessarily all dire, you can manage kidney disease and slow the progression by eating nutritious foods, taking your meds, exercising on a regular basis, and following up with your medical provider.

In spite of my many medical conditions, I remain positive and surround myself with loving and supportive family and friends. Sometimes, it is difficult to do, but I attempt to exercise daily, along with receiving encouragement from my friends.

I truly miss my mother and sister and look forward to seeing them again when the time is right. My immediate family mostly lives in the South now—Charlotte, North Carolina, and Memphis, Tennessee. The Lord has blessed me with being a mother, grandmother, niece, cousin, aunt, great-aunt, great-great aunt, and a great-great-great aunt to a host of nieces and nephews. I feel truly blessed.

Also, I would love to become a motivational speaker to senior citizens at senior facilities such as residential, nursing homes, or community-based locations. I would enjoy getting the opportunity to speak to seniors sixty-five and older to tell them about my experiences—personal and medically related—and answer any questions they may have along with motivating and encouraging them to remain positive regarding any medical ailments or personal problems they may have, such as losing loved ones, or any goals, aspirations, or endeavors they would still like to pursue.

I will continue to meditate, pray and be positive. As I said at the beginning of my story, in spite of my many chronic ailments and medical conditions, I am the healthiest sick person I know.

Thank you, dear God.

ABOUT THE AUTHOR

Marsha Nixon Powell is a Philadelphia native. She lives with her family in Northeast Philadelphia. She is a longtime cancer survivor who has been a business owner and currently works as a behavioral health technician in the Philadelphia school system with autistic and special-needs students.

She also works as a home caregiver for senior citizens in the Philadelphia and Bucks County areas. She is an inspiration to those who know her and continues to learn and develop new leadership and professional skills.

Marsha is a hard worker, and in spite of her many ailments and chronic conditions, she is still going strong at seventy-four years of age!

Printed in the USA
CPSIA information can be obtained
at www.ICGtesting.com
LVHW011640130624
782911LV00003B/477